50 THINGS TO KNOW
BOOK SERIES
REVIEWS FROM READERS

I recently downloaded a couple of books from this series to read over the weekend thinking I would read just one or two. However, I so loved the books that I read all the six books I had downloaded in one go and ended up downloading a few more today. Written by different authors, the books offer practical advice on how you can perform or achieve certain goals in life, which in this case is how to have a better life.

The information is simple to digest and learn from, and is incredibly useful. There are also resources listed at the end of the book that you can use to get more information.

50 Things To Know To Have A Better Life: Self-Improvement Made Easy! by Dannii Cohen

---

This book is very helpful and provides simple tips on how to improve your everyday life. I found it to be useful in improving my overall attitude.

50 Things to Know For Your Mindfulness & Meditation Journey by Nina Edmondso

---

Quick read with 50 short and easy tips for what to think about before starting to homeschool.

50 Things to Know About Getting Started with Homeschool by Amanda Walton

i

50 Things to Know

I really enjoyed the voice of the narrator, she speaks in a soothing tone. The book is a really great reminder of things we might have known we could do during stressful times, but forgot over the years.

- HarmonyHawaii

50 Things to Know to Manage Your Stress: Relieve The Pressure and Return The Joy To Your Life

by Diane Whitbeck

There is so much waste in our society today. Everyone should be forced to read this book. I know I am passing it on to my family.

50 Things to Know to Downsize Your Life: How To Downsize, Organize, And Get Back to Basics

by Lisa Rusczyk Ed. D.

Great book to get you motivated and understand why you may be losing motivation. Great for that person who wants to start getting healthy, or just for you when you need motivation while having an established workout routine.

50 Things To Know To Stick With A Workout: Motivational Tips To Start The New You Today

by Sarah Hughes

50 THINGS TO KNOW ABOUT CHRONIC ILLNESS

Mara Price-Quinn

50 Things to Know

Cover designed by: Ivana Stamenkovic
Cover Image: https://pixabay.com/en/computer-business-office-technology-3343887/

Edited by:

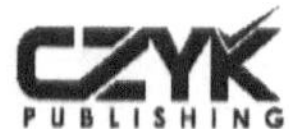

CZYK Publishing Since 2011.

50 Things to Know
Visit our website at www.50thingstoknow..com

Lock Haven, PA

ISBN: 9781723864773

50 THINGS TO KNOW ABOUT CHRONIC ILLNESS

BOOK DESCRIPTION

Have you just been diagnosed with a chronic illness, and you don't know where to turn? Or, perhaps, someone close to you has just received a diagnosis, and you would like to learn how to support them in their chronic illness journey. Either way, this book is for you! 50 Things to Know About Chronic Illness by Mara Price-Quinn offers 50 great tips on how to deal with your chronic illness or how to help and support your loved ones who deal with chronic illness. You can hear what it is like to experience a chronic illness from someone who has a chronic illness herself and find ways to improve your quality of life, no matter how you're feeling. Hopefully by the end, you will feel more empowered in your chronic illness journey.

TABLE OF CONTENTS

DEDICATION

This book is dedicated to my mom, Cheryl. Mom, from the very first, you taught me how to be an advocate for my health. You have had to be persistent in making sure you received the best treatment, and I hope I have taken a page out of your book in doing the same. Your illness never got in the way of being a great parent, even on your worst days, and I truly want to thank you for that. You and Dad taught me to be a strong person, no matter what life throws at me, and I am so grateful to have had you there for me in my own chronic illness journey. Thank you for all that you do! I love you!

ABOUT THE AUTHOR

Mara Price-Quinn has been a writer for as long as she can remember. She is an accomplished poet; she participated in the Gilbert Chappell Distinguished Poet Series, won several awards for her poetry, and was published in college journals and in a volume of poetry from North Carolina writers. She also enjoys writing fiction and nonfiction, and her love of the written word also extends to editing and tutoring. As a tutor, she has helped everyone from kindergarteners to adults returning to school.

After graduating in 2017 with degrees in English and psychology, Mara took a gap year to get married, work, and have time to herself. She has worked as an after-school teacher and a transcriber, and also makes crafts to sell in her free time. Aside from writing, she enjoys spending time with loved ones, reading, listening to music, watching horror movies, sewing, weaving, pottery, painting, singing, cooking with her husband, and hanging out with her beloved beagle, Waffles. She is currently pursuing a career as a paralegal, and has plans to go back to school someday.

Her own chronic illness journey began at birth: she was diagnosed with asthma, which still persists today.

In high school, she was diagnosed with Hashimoto's thyroiditis, an autoimmune disorder that affects her thyroid and causes symptoms like migraines, fatigue, insomnia, mood swings, and chronic pain. With the help of her doctors and her loved ones, she works hard to maintain her physical and mental health and advocate for others who are ill. She enjoys her life, and is happier today than she was before she was ever diagnosed... though it would be nice to not have to deal with Hashimoto's anymore!

1. LEARN ABOUT YOUR DIAGNOSIS

So, you've been diagnosed with a chronic illness. This could mean you have anything from arthritis to schizophrenia - chronic illnesses can affect any part of your body or mental state. The prognosis for your chronic illness may look very different from someone else's, and even if you have the same chronic illness as someone else, it doesn't mean it will affect you the same way. The first step to take when you receive your diagnosis is ask questions about it and do some research of your own.

And I don't just mean googling it and reading a couple of articles online; try to get in contact with real people who have the same illness, or have a good conversation with your doctor or a specialist about what your diagnosis means. Remember, though, people with the same illness can often experience different symptoms, so one person's story does not apply to everyone with the same illness. It is important to gain information from lots of credible sources. And if you have access to any kind of research database – say, if you are a student and your school has an extensive library – try looking up your disease sometime. You may be surprised with the amount of information there is about it.

2. GET READY FOR LOTS OF UNSOLICITED ADVICE

If you tell your friends and family about your diagnosis, prepare yourself for an influx of tips and tricks that you didn't ask for. One friend might suggest you start taking a new vitamin supplement, while a coworker will tell you about how going gluten free fixed all of her problems. Now, these suggestions may be made with the best intentions, and they may really work for people. But you need to take charge of your own health and decide what you will and will not do. And if the unsolicited advice becomes too much, don't be afraid to tell your loved ones to back off a little. Even if you're a non-confrontational person, like me, you will thank yourself for it in the end. Your chronic illness journey is yours, and you get to choose who has a say in it.

3. LEARN TO DISTINGUISH BETWEEN SCIENCE AND PSEUDOSCIENCE

There is a lot of information out there today, and not all of it is trustworthy. In the age of the Internet, anyone can say anything, and you want to make sure you're getting your information from reputable sources. And don't be afraid to ask your doctor about something you've read or heard from someone else - they will very likely be able to confirm or deny the claim! If you have a good doctor who is familiar with your illnesses and is understanding, you should trust in what they say than a blogger on an Internet who has a degree in gaining followers.

4. BE ASSERTIVE AT THE DOCTOR'S OFFICE

You know that your headaches haven't gotten better. You have been dealing with indigestion for weeks. The cramps you have once a month are worse than they ever have been. Don't beat around the bush when you're sitting on the exam table. Your doctor is not there to judge you, they are there to treat you, and that means treating all of you. If you open up more about the symptoms you are experiencing, you could potentially find answers for why they are so severe or bothersome. Your doctor can discern whether the medications you are on are the right ones for you, or decide a new prescription would be beneficial. Either way, there is nothing to be lost from being more up front about your symptoms. Even if the details are "embarrassing," don't worry. Doctors really have heard it all!

5. LISTEN TO YOUR BODY AND LEARN YOUR SYMPTOMS

When you are first diagnosed with a chronic illness, it may be hard to tell what's a symptom and what's a normal bodily function. You may be out of breath after going for a brisk run, which would generally be a normal symptom to have, or you may be out of breath sitting at your computer desk, due to your asthma. These symptoms are not the same. Learning how your chronic illness affects your body specifically can help you to rule out what is normal and what is not, and when you should talk to your doctor about making medication changes or finding other methods of treatment.

6. LOOK INTO MAKING DIET CHANGES

Say you've just been diagnosed with diabetes or an eating disorder. These conditions will likely require changes to your diet. Seeing a nutritionist and receiving some information about the caloric and nutritional needs your body has can be really helpful in your journey with chronic illness. Diet changes certainly are not going to cure you, and when all is said and done, they may not affect you that much; however, if there is any chance that they could help you, it is worth trying.

7. TAKE CARE OF YOURSELF MENTALLY

Perhaps your chronic illness primarily affects your mental state. Or, maybe, the effects your chronic illness is having on your body is taking a toll on you emotionally. If either is the case, you should look into receiving the proper care for yourself mentally. Remember: mental health is just as important as physical health, and the two often go hand in hand! If you are not feeling well physically, it will very likely affect your mood. There is no shame in seeking out a therapist, taking medication for mental conditions, or even just reaching out to a trusted friend or family member to discuss your state of mind.

8. DON'T PUSH YOURSELF TOO HARD

Oftentimes, living with a chronic illness means your limits will be different than others' limits. Say your roommate may be able to run a mile every morning, but doing so makes your joints ache or your lungs struggle for air. Don't feel like you have to be at their level. Find an exercise routine that works for you. Remember to take frequent breaks and check in on your body.

Additionally, you may find that your mental limits may be lower than other people's. If you find large social events exhausting due to chronic fatigue, or your insomnia prevents you from meeting an early deadline, don't be afraid to decline invitations or ask for more time. I am sure you know that sometimes in life we don't get second chances or extra time for important projects, but there is no harm in asking. And you never know, the friends or supervisors that you have could be more understanding than you think.

9. FIND A SUPPORT GROUP

There are many groups out there for people with all sorts of chronic illnesses. Even if your illness is on the rarer side, you can likely still find a group on Facebook or similar social media sites that will apply to you. These groups can be a great source of support, and you may find the answers to questions you've been having about your illness. You could even make some new friends along the way who truly understand your journey with chronic illness. Support groups are a great way to feel less alone, which is something everyone needs.

Again, though, remember that not everyone with the same illness experiences the same symptoms, or is helped by the same treatment. I know people who have the same illness that I do that have completely different side effects on one medication that I have on the same medication. There usually a "one size fits all" pill or therapy. Still, support groups have helped me a lot in gaining information and trying new things that have actually helped me in many ways.

10. PRIORITIZE SLEEP

Sleep is when the body repairs itself! Taking steps to ensure that you are getting enough sleep at night is extremely important. A healthy sleep schedule will make you feel better physically and mentally. As long as you get at least eight hours - and you may need more, especially on days where your symptoms are severe - you will see a difference in how you feel. Try going to bed at the same time every night and waking up around the same time each day.

Prioritizing sleep can influence your life in ways that may be difficult to adjust to. If you are a night owl, you may find it hard to fall asleep at a reasonable time and not oversleep during the day. If you are used to hanging out with friends late into the night, or hanging out with them so often that you don't have much time to sleep, tell them that you have to leave by a certain time. You don't even have to explain why you're heading home; if your friends care about you, they will understand. Sleep is vital to a healthy life, and prioritizing it will go a long way in making you feel better.

Your sleep can also be affected by factors like your mattress, the positions you sleep in, your pillows, whether you sleep with the TV on, what you eat before bed... you get the idea! If you are a coffee or soda drinker, make sure to set a strict cut-off time for caffeine so you can get to sleep at a reasonable time. Even if you are a student, try not to pull all-nighters; studies show that cramming all night and not sleeping can be detrimental to your grades. And if you find yourself falling asleep with the TV on every night, try falling asleep to it at a lower volume or turning it off altogether and playing some calming music or white noise. If you examine your sleeping habits, you may find ways to improve your sleep and, in turn, your overall health.

11. STAY ON TOP OF YOUR SCHEDULE

Trying to fit five doctor's appointments into your calendar is hard work. I find that setting multiple reminders on my phone helps me a lot. Basically, if it isn't in my phone, it doesn't exist. You may find that this method works for you, or you might try something different, like putting your schedule on your fridge or using a dry erase board. Do whatever you can to help you remember your appointments, and try to record everything so you know exactly where you'll be and when. This will make it a lot easier when you are trying to fit something else in, like fun times with friends or a date you've been trying to plan for weeks.

12. DO THINGS THAT MAKE YOU FEEL GOOD

This is a good tip for everyone, but especially for those who deal daily with the realities of chronic illness. Some days, my illnesses just make me feel like crap! And on those days, I try to do things that relax me and make me feel better. Some days, that's marathoning a show on TV, or sharing a bottle of wine with a good friend. These things may not be considered "healthy," but if they make you feel better, even in the short term, they have value. Life is not all about doing the right thing all of the time.

13. DON'T BE AFRAID TO HAVE A LAZY DAY

This kind of goes along with #12. You're a hardworking person, and you feel guilty whenever you spend too long on the couch or eat too much without exercising. But here's the reality: chronic illnesses are exhausting. Even if your illness is not specifically chronic fatigue, or even if that isn't one of the symptoms, it is still a tiring job trying to maintain control of your health. Everyone needs a day where they can unwind and do nothing – even people without chronic illness!

That being said, I am not advocating that you don't take care of yourself! Just the opposite. Many cultures recognize the importance of having a "lazy day," or simply doing things that are an indulgence rather than a need. We can't live our lives constantly trying to meet a certain standard. On our especially bad days, we need to have that something we can turn to that just makes us feel like us again. And whatever that is for you, as long as it isn't actively making your illnesses worse, you should take the time to treat yourself.

14. PRACTICE POSITIVITY

It may seem cheesy, but changing up negative thought patterns can go a long way in making you feel better. We can all think ourselves into a "thought spiral" at times – I know that is definitely true for me. But with the help of my therapist, I have been able to challenge some of those negative thoughts that work so hard to bring me down. I would have so many days where I just couldn't leave my bed or do anything productive because I just felt like it wouldn't be worth anything anyways.

But when I started examining my thought patterns more thoroughly, I began to notice the fallacies in logic and the way they were truly bringing me down. And if you have your mind constantly trying to bring you down, how do you think that is going to affect your body? They are certainly connected! So if you, too, struggle with self-defeating thought patterns, seek the help of a therapist or a good friend, or maybe even read up on a couple of self-help books to help you combat that little voice of negativity that's constantly nagging at you. It can go a long way in improving your overall health.

15. BUT, DON'T BE AFRAID TO FEEL NEGATIVE EMOTIONS

When you're first diagnosed, you may feel that you are experiencing the first five stages of grief. In a moment, your life has changed, and now you have to alter the way you live. This will bring up emotions like anger, sadness, and frustration - and that's okay! These are normal responses to a major life change, like unfortunate medical news. Don't try to minimize your feelings or pretend like everything is okay - it will be better for you in the long run to acknowledge your emotions and discuss them with loved ones or a professional.

And it's so important to express your feelings! If you are artistic, maybe you find a lot of catharsis in creating something out of your pain. Or perhaps you find more comfort in sharing with a loved one. However that expression may take form, it is widely known that letting it out in some way is much better than bottling it up.

16. TAKE CARE OF YOUR IMMUNE SYSTEM

I have had asthma for my whole life, and asthma makes my lungs more susceptible to infection. I get bronchitis at least once a year, and it has lead to several visits to the ER. This bronchitis can last for weeks, and it's awful. However, I have learned that there are certain things I need to avoid to minimize my chance of picking up bronchitis. For example, when I worked with kids, I found myself getting sick a lot more often (seems like a no-brainer, right?). Traveling can also trigger my bronchitis, especially if I travel somewhere with unfamiliar allergens, like the mountains.

So, when I do have to interact with a lot of kids, or if I am traveling somewhere, I take precautions to minimize my chances of an asthma flare up. I always bring my rescue inhaler, Germ-X my hands often, take over-the-counter allergy medications, or sanitize surfaces that many people have touched. I also do simple things like making sure I get enough sleep, drink enough water, and have enough vitamin C. These practices may seem finicky, but my health is worth being finicky over. Take care of your immune system as best as you can, and you may see a difference in how often you get really sick.

17. LEARN YOUR TRIGGERS

You may find that your chronic pain is worse after an intense period of exercise. Or that exposure to lots of loud noise triggers your migraines. Either way, try to take note of when you experience symptoms. This can be made easier by journaling, which I will write about in more detail later on. Figuring out what your triggers are can be an important step in coping with your chronic illness.

18. EXAMINE YOUR HABITS

When you're sitting at your desk at work, how is your posture? How much screen time are you spending in your life outside of work? Are you taking enough breaks for stretching or sitting? Are you eating and drinking water often enough? It may not seem like much, but these elements can add up to either worsen or improve your chronic illness. Keeping good posture can ease arthritis or back pain, and reducing screen time might help your headaches. Stretching after long periods of sitting down, or sitting after long periods of standing, will ease tension in your muscles. Staying hydrated and not going hungry will always make you feel better.

19. BE GUNG-HO ABOUT TAKING MEDICATION

It's hard to incorporate new medications into your already hectic routine. But it's important that you take them on a consistent basis for them to take full effect. Try setting reminders on your phone if you have a hard time remembering when to take them, or purchase a pill box if you have multiple prescriptions and forget to take one. If you are going to be somewhere during the time you normally take your medication, make sure to bring your prescriptions with you, and perhaps a bottle of water if you need.

Be watchful about what can interact with your medications, and how they affect you and your functioning. If you have a medication that interacts with alcohol to make you drowsy, limit your intake of alcohol or at least make sure you have a reliable way of getting home in the event you are too sleepy to drive, even if you just have one glass of wine. Read the labels on over-the-counter medications to make sure they can be taken with your prescription medications, and don't be afraid to call your pharmacist if you have any questions. It is better to know than to not be sure and have something bad happen as a result of not knowing.

You should also monitor the side effects your medications have on you. The same prescription can affect two people very differently, so don't think that just because someone else has nausea on one medication, that you will automatically get nausea. Stay abreast of what side effects are considered "normal" versus the side effects that are rare. And remember it takes a few weeks to get used to some prescriptions; when I first started my Zoloft prescription, for example, I dealt with nausea for about a week before I got used to it. And don't be afraid to ask your doctor what other medication options you have if your side effects are particularly bad. If it seems to be helping with your chronic illness, but giving you terrible migraine headaches, maybe it is not the right medication for you!

20. PURSUE EMPLOYMENT THAT WORKS FOR YOU

If your chronic illness makes it difficult to be at work for eight hours a day, maybe it's time to start looking for a new job. Today, there are many career opportunities you can pursue from your own home. I found that transcribing helped me make money while not exacerbating the symptoms of my chronic illness, and I could go to my appointments without having to call out of work. There are other flexible jobs you could pursue outside of your home, or you could simply look for a job that won't make the symptoms of your illnesses worse. For example, if you find it difficult to be on your feet for long hours, or doing hard manual labor, perhaps you shouldn't look for jobs where you will need to perform these duties. Either way, if you can, you should try to make sure you find a job that works for your and your health.

21. IF YOU CANNOT FIND EMPLOYMENT THAT BETTER SUITS YOUR NEEDS, REACH OUT TO YOUR BOSSES AND SEE IF ACCOMMODATIONS CAN BE MADE

Perhaps you will find that some, but not all, of your work can be done at home, and you only need to go to the office three or four days a week instead of five. Or, perhaps you can bring certain items into the workplace that help you manage your symptoms, like heating pads. Maybe your boss can get some blackout curtains for your office window so that your migraines are not as bad, or you can see about ordering a chair with better lumbar support so your chronic pain isn't beating you up at the end of the day.

If you have an understanding work environment, don't be afraid to ask for what would help you feel better. Work is a huge part of our lives, and no one deserves to have their chronic illness symptoms worsened by the way they are working. Good supervisors will look for ways to help you feel better, because it not only helps you, it can also help them in their business, too! Happy employees makes for a happy company.

22. EXAMINE YOUR ENVIRONMENT

When I discovered that I had a dust allergy that worsens my asthma symptoms, I had to examine my environment pretty thoroughly. This involves washing my sheets on a more frequent basis than other people, and making sure my surroundings are clean as well as I can. These changes to my environment make it so my allergies are not as bad, and in turn, they do not trigger my asthma as badly or as often.

For you, this may look different. There are many environmental factors that can affect the way you feel. Stairs, for example, can be a big trigger for chronic pain. If you live somewhere with stairs, try to minimize the times you have to go up and down them. This may involve making sure you have everything you need before heading upstairs, and vice versa. Or, you may find that the noise levels you are exposed to trigger your migraines. If there are ways you can reduce the noise levels you are exposed to, take those measures. You can even purchase noise-canceling headphones if you have noisy neighbors or if small sounds are irritating when you have a migraine.

Whatever your chronic illness is, examining your environment can go a long way in reducing your pain levels and making you feel better overall. Finding little ways to improve your environment may make your chronic illness feel much more manageable. Hopefully, you can find any environmental triggers you may have and take the steps you need to take to change them.

23. PUT TOGETHER YOUR OWN "TOOLBOX" FOR DAYS WHEN YOU ARE FEELING PARTICULARLY

UNWELL

On your particularly bad days, keep a stash of supplies that will help you to feel better. This could mean a multitude of things: maybe having some chocolate helps when your chronic pain is severe, or maybe having a glass of wine and taking a bubble bath helps soothe your sore muscles. Make sure you keep these items that make you feel better in your house so that you can access them when you really need them. And even if these items make you feel better "superficially," try not to feel ashamed for indulging when you are exhausted and in pain. If it makes you feel better, it makes you feel better, and that matters.

24. BE PROACTIVE

If you start noticing a new or worsening symptom, don't wait too long to make an appointment! There is a difference between being a hypochondriac and being proactive about your health. If your knee has started to ache with any physical activity that you do, try getting in to see a physical therapist. If your depressive episode starts worsening to the point where you are unable to function at all, reach out to a psychiatrist. It can take a long time to get in to see your doctor, and potentially even longer to see a specialist, so try to schedule your appointments before your symptoms get unbearable.

25. SURROUND YOURSELF WITH PEOPLE WHO UNDERSTAND

Whether this involves joining a support group or simply making new friends that are understanding of your chronic illness, having a community of people you can count on is important. If someone is constantly putting you down because of your chronic illness, or the limitations it presents, don't be afraid of minimizing your interactions with them! Negative influences don't do any good for your wellbeing, physical or otherwise.

Your support group can of course also include your therapist and doctor/doctors. The specialists you choose to give your money to and who you choose to help you treat your illness should be understanding and caring. I'm not saying you have to be best friends, but they need to be sympathetic to your needs and listen to you when you have concerns. If you feel like any of your doctor/patient relationships are not healthy, you should discontinue those relationships and seek out other specialists to go to instead. Your chronic illness journey is going to stick with you a lot longer than any doctor will, most likely, so you need to choose people who will be helpful to you as you walk through it.

26. REMEMBER, NOT ALL ILLNESSES ARE VISIBLE

Just because someone is smiling does not mean that everything is okay and that they are feeling well. People with chronic illness are good at putting on a mask when they are around others. This may be because they do not want others to know how they are really feeling, or it could simply be because they genuinely are feeling okay in that moment, and their symptoms are manageable. But that does not mean they aren't struggling or are feeling up to do anything.

I am sure you have heard the old quote attributed to Plato: "Be kind, for everyone you meet is fighting a hard battle." That quote may be a bit overused, but it does have some value. People with chronic illnesses may not only be fighting a hard battle, they may be fighting an invisible battle. They may feel pressured by society to put on that happy face and act like everything is okay, when things are just the opposite. So be kind, and believe people when they tell you they are unable to do something or they don't feel up to hanging out. It may not be obvious to you, but their chronic illness may be preventing them from doing things with you.

27. JOURNALING CAN HELP IN MULTIPLE WAYS

If you already like to journal, you might find it easy to keep a journal for your chronic illness journey. Journaling can be helpful in several ways: they can keep track of your symptoms, point out potential triggers for things like migraines or chronic pain, and monitor whether a new medication seems to be improving your condition or not.

Keeping track of your symptoms can be made easier by keeping a journal. Many people who experience migraines, for example, keep a migraine journal. This can help them determine whether their symptoms seem to be worsening, or whether their migraines are lasting longer or are more easily triggered. Journals like this are also great to bring into your doctor to help you remember exactly what's been going on and provide some evidence as to the severity and frequency of your symptoms.

Today, there are many creative and even fun ways to journal, so don't think that journaling about illness needs to be boring and dry. Even if you are not the best at journaling or being creative, there are tutorials for "bullet journals" online and other ways you can make your journaling experience more enjoyable. Making time to journal each day can be extremely helpful in helping manage your chronic illness.

28. LOOK INTO SEEING A SPECIALIST

Maybe you've been seeing your general practitioner since you were a kid. Now, all of a sudden, you've got a chronic illness. While your GP may be well equipped to run tests and prescribe medication for your condition, they may not be specifically trained in the disease that you have. If you have a thyroid condition, look into endocrinologists in your area. If your illness affects the quality of your skin, seek out a dermatologist.

These professionals may have the specialized knowledge you need to help you in your journey with chronic illness.

Don't be afraid that you may "offend" your doctor by seeing another specialist. This is certainly not the case! If your doctor is supportive of you in your chronic illness journey, they will be more than happy to send any medical records to the way of your specialist. A good doctor wants to help you succeed, not hold you back from success.

29. DON'T READ TOO MUCH ONLINE

If you're a frequent symptom checker, you may continuously believe you've got brain cancer when you have a headache. While there is a lot of great information out there on the Internet, you can also become too inundated with stories from others about the illness you may have; remember, people often experience different symptoms and issues, even with the same illness. If you are worried about something, step away from the keyboard for a bit and call your doctor to make an appointment.

Additionally, we all know that reading the comments on certain articles can never yield good results. If you read articles about chronic illness, try to refrain from reading the comment sections; they can often hide comments from people who believe very negative things about people with chronic illnesses. Exposing yourself to these toxic ways of thinking won't do anything for you. And try not to engage in people online who just want to be trolls; there is a time and place to share your experiences, certainly, but some people simply can't be reasoned with, and you shouldn't have to waste your time and energy on people who are just trying to get a rise out of you.

30. LOOK FOR SMALL, INEXPENSIVE THINGS TO HELP YOU ON A DAY-TO-DAY BASIS

This may mean investing in a heating pad to help with chronic pain, or purchasing a pill organizer for the different medications you have to take in a day. If it makes dealing with your chronic illness easier, it's worth it. You shouldn't have to feel bad for using things that make your life easier and your chronic illness more manageable.

Many people are familiar with informercials, and the way that the actors in them overexaggerate to an almost comical level. However, the products in these commercials are often geared towards people with disabilities. The next time you see one of these commercials, try to see how the product can help people who have difficulty performing a certain task. You may find that the product in question would help you in one of your daily activities that you have a hard time with.

31. DON'T TAKE ANYBODY'S BS

Just like there is stigma surrounding mental illness, there is a lot of stigma out there about chronic illness. As terrible as it sounds, there are people who believe that chronically ill people are "making it all up" for attention. Or, perhaps, they believe that people should "just get over it." And you may come across this rhetoric in your chronic illness journey, whether in real life or online.

People tend to be more bold online, where things are relatively anonymous and they are detached from the emotional impact that their words can have. I'm sure you are familiar with all of the "trolls" that get a kick out of being cruel to others under the cover of a faceless social media account. But here's the thing: you don't have to engage with them. In fact, it can be more exhausting to argue with them, as they don't care about changing their mind; they just want to get a rise out of people. The next time you see someone trying to stir the pot and insulting people with chronic illness, examine whether you have the mental energy to engage. If not, just block the person and move on.

Dealing with loved ones is hopefully different. You may come across some friends or relatives who are not informed about the realities of chronic illness, and who can say some ignorant or inconsiderate things. Hopefully, you are at a point in your relationship with them where you can point out why the things they are saying are wrong, and maybe even explaining why. However, even when it comes to people in real life, you still don't need to feel like it is your responsibility to educate others, or constantly argue in defense of your chronic illness journey. You don't need to rely on others' validation of your illness to make it "real." You know how real it is, you deal with it every day! So, if these conversations ever reach a point where you are getting emotionally exhausted with little to no positive results, don't be afraid to stay away and limit your contact with these people.

32. YOU MAY NOT BE ABLE TO DO THE SAME THINGS THAT YOU USED TO DO, AND THAT'S OKAY

Maybe you used to go to the gym five times a week, and since your diagnosis, you've found that you can only manage a couple days a week, if at all. That's okay. You may find that you aren't able to have the same routine that you used to have before dealing with your symptoms.

You may find this adjustment to be very difficult, and that's also okay. It can feel very discouraging to not be able to do the things you used to do. However, you may still be able to enjoy these activities in moderation, or even different activities that you can do instead. You don't have to be the same person for forever; people change, and there's nothing wrong with that.

33. FIND A DOCTOR WHO LISTENS

This might seem like a no-brainer, but this is hugely important in coping with your chronic illness. Sympathetic doctors can make everything so much easier, even if it just makes you feel better emotionally. You should feel comfortable enough with your doctor that you are able to talk about all of your symptoms and concerns. You should feel confident in their recommendations for treating your chronic illness. If these things don't apply, it may be time to look for a new doctor.

34. DON'T COMPARE YOUR DIFFICULTIES TO OTHERS' DIFFICULTIES

Everyone is fighting their own battles. Cliché, right? But we all certainly know it to be true. You may have a chronic illness that does not affect your life on a day to day basis, and in comparison to others' experiences with chronic illness, you may feel like you don't "deserve" to complain or take a day off. But chronic illness takes many forms, and it's very rarely smooth sailing. Even if your illness affects you in less visible or extreme ways that other people are affected, your experience is still valid, and you still deserve to take care of yourself.

35. BE ASSERTIVE IN YOUR PERSONAL LIFE

Don't be afraid to ask for what you need. If the party you're at is wiping you out, and you don't feel like going out for drinks afterwards, say so. If you need help putting the dishes away at night, don't be afraid to ask your partner for some help. Being assertive in your personal life about your limitations and needs will help you out in the long run, and your true friends and loved ones will be happy to help you in any way they can. I have found that my friends are very understanding of when I just don't feel well or have had too much social time, and no one has helped me more than my husband. If I don't feel like going somewhere or doing a task that I normally would be fine doing, he is more than happy to step in and help me out, or give me some alone time if I need it. Being assertive has helped me manage my symptoms and chronic illness better than if I forced myself to do things that made my symptoms worse.

36. FIND A PHARMACY THAT WORKS FOR YOU

Your doctor will not be the only health professional you will deal with in your chronic illness journey. You will likely receive a medication from your doctor, and perhaps more than one. If you don't already go to a pharmacist on a regular basis, do some research to see what the best pharmacist for you would be. Find a convenient location to your home or workplace so you can pick up your prescriptions at the best time for you. If a certain pharmacist seems to have a bad attitude, or if the pharmacy itself doesn't seem to be efficiently run, move on. If you're interested in automatic refills, see if your pharmacy can do that for you. In the end, you should have a pharmacy that works for you.

37. CUT DOWN ON ERRANDS THAT TIRE YOU OUT BY TURNING TO THE INTERNET

Today, food delivery services are more accessible and affordable than ever. If you find it difficult to get to the store on some days, or if you have a hard time cooking, look into a food delivery service. Today there are options to order all of your groceries online and either drive up to the store to pick them up or have them delivered to your residence. There may be an extra fee involved for delivery or pickup services, but there may not be! Do some research into what could be the best option for you.

Meal delivery services have also grown in popularity. Today there are several to choose from, with different options for people with food allergies or dietary restrictions. They can also make it easier to cook healthier food without having to plan out a recipe or go to the store, things that can take a lot of time and energy. If this sounds like a good option for you, check out the different brands and price options; you may be surprised how much it can help.

38. WHEN YOU ARE AWAY FROM HOME, BRING ANY EMERGENCY SUPPLIES YOU MAY NEED

This may seem like a no-brainer, but when you are first diagnosed, it can be very difficult to remember to always have your EpiPen or pain medications on hand. If you know you are going somewhere, prepare ahead of time by putting your medications or enough of a dosage into your bag or car so that you won't have to worry about turning around once you're on the road. However, make sure that you are storing your medication properly; for example, EpiPens need to be stored at certain temperatures, so you can't keep them in your car on a hot summer day. Either way, double checking to make sure you've got your medications – over-the-counter or otherwise – can help you to feel good even when you're away from home.

If you need to bring something other than medication, like a list of your medications or your insurance card for emergencies, you should also make sure to pack those ahead of time. Making sure your phone is fully charged is also very helpful if you need help but aren't at home. Whatever supplies you rely on from a day-to-day basis should be on hand even when your routine changes.

39. WHEN YOU ARE PACKING FOR A TRIP, MAKE SURE YOU WON'T NEED ANY REFILLS BEFORE YOU

COME HOME

This is another simple tip that may seem like a given, but when you are packing in a rush, it can be easy to forget whether you have enough medication to get you through. If you are running low, it would be a good idea to call in a refill to pick up before you go or to have ready when you get back. It is also smart to remember to bring a list of medications and a copy of your insurance just in case you run into any emergencies.

40. CONSIDER WHETHER THE TIME COMMITMENTS YOU MAKE ARE FEASIBLE FOR YOU

If you're joining a book club or an exercise group or anything else that requires recurring social events, evaluate whether you will be able to keep up with the meetings or tasks that these groups involve. I certainly recommend joining social groups, but people with chronic illnesses may have less energy or may not be able to foretell how much time they will be able to dedicate to frequent meetings. Hopefully, you join groups with members that are understanding and supportive of your chronic illness journey, but if your particular group requires strict attendance or specific tasks that require a lot of your time and energy, they might not be the right group for your needs.

For example, I am a member of a movie and music club with a couple of friends. Because we all live in different cities, our interactions take place online over a group chat. Every week, someone in our group picks out a movie to watch or an album to listen to, and when everyone has watched or listened to the movie or album, we discuss it in detail. This is a pretty easy group to keep up with when it's online, and movies and music are more accessible than ever. However, even in this group, there are times where someone has to take a week off or simply can't listen to a certain album or watch a certain movie. And thankfully, my friends are very understanding and adjust accordingly whenever someone needs a break. So even low-maintenance, online groups can take up some of your time and energy when you are dealing with chronic illness.

41. YOU DON'T HAVE TO SUFFER IN

I have personally found that being vocal about my chronic illness journey has helped me to feel less alone. By speaking out, I've discovered new friends that deal with chronic illness, and even friends I already had that had been dealing with chronic illness but were afraid to be open about it. Either way, for me personally, speaking out into the void helps me a lot.

That may not be the same case for you, but you may still find comfort in confiding with a friend or close family member about your chronic illness. If you have someone you really trust, try discussing how you feel and see how it goes. Hopefully your loved one will be a good listening ear, and they will be there for you whenever you want to talk about anything related to chronic illness.

42. REMEMBER THAT IT ISN'T YOUR FAULT THAT YOU HAVE A CHRONIC ILLNESS

Dealing with chronic illness, especially when it triggers a depression, can involve lots of feelings of shame and guilt. You may feel like your diet or activity level has caused you to have a chronic illness. And even if your illness is related to those things, whether or not you get a chronic illness is dependent on many different factors. Genetics can certainly play a part in whether you get a chronic illness or not, and genetics is not exactly something you can control. Additionally, not all people with poor diets and poor activity levels get diagnosed with a chronic illness. So if it was all dependent upon your diet or activity level, everyone with the same behaviors would experience the same issues. Some factors are simply out of your control.

Furthermore, you may even be tempted to think that you deserve to have a chronic illness, especially if you have not "taken care of your body." That is certainly not the case. Many factors contribute to poor diet and poor activity levels, for example, not just laziness or apathy. For example, people often fail to consider how much easier and cheaper it is to buy unhealthy food. And when you don't have much money or much time to buy and cook healthier meals, junk food is your main option.

I am not suggesting that people don't take responsibility for their choices. We do have some responsibility over our health and livelihoods. But

sometimes things simply spiral out of our control.
And even if we "caused" our chronic illness in one
way or another, it doesn't mean that our diagnoses are
our punishments.

43. YOUR PAIN IS VALID, AND NOT ALL IN YOUR HEAD

Don't fool yourself into thinking this is something
you can just get over or that you are making a big
deal over nothing. Chronic illness is no joke. It can be
extremely difficult to deal with on a day to day basis.
You know the symptoms you experience and how
they affect your life; even if the people around you
don't believe you or minimize your experience, that
experience is still valid.

I was diagnosed with my thyroid condition over
six years ago, and I still experience a lot of doubt
about my illness. I second guess whether a symptom I
am having is something I should make a big deal out
of. I have a hard time determining whether I'm just
tired, or whether my thyroid is not functioning well.
And this can make it feel like I am making it all up or
exaggerating my symptoms – even though I have a
doctor's diagnosis! Those little thoughts of self-doubt

may never leave your mind, but try to remember that what you are experiencing is not simply something you made up.

44. YOU DON'T HAVE TO BE YOUR FRIENDS' SOURCE OF INFORMATION ABOUT YOUR ILLNESS OR ILLNESS IN GENERAL

When I was diagnosed with my thyroid condition, a dear friend of mine began to worry that they might have the same condition. They would tell me about all of their symptoms, and ask me if I thought they had the same illness. Now, I love this friend, but this behavior honestly irritated me a bit. Firstly, their symptoms did not seem out of the ordinary for any human to experience: an occasional headache, or some general tiredness, does not immediately indicate something is wrong with your thyroid! And secondly, my only suggestion for that friend was to go to the doctor if they were concerned. Just because I have this condition does not mean I'm an expert on it! And that's not even to mention how people with the same condition can experience a vast array of symptoms, and other diseases can also cause similar symptoms.

So if you find that your friends or family members are pestering you more often about their own health concerns, try not to engage. Keep your responses minimal, be direct and firm, and always recommend them to see a doctor if they are truly concerned.

45. TAKE YOUR TIME TO RECOVER

Chronic illness is exhausting, and on top of that, your body may take longer to recover than people who do not experience chronic illness. If you go to a particularly exhausting social outing, or if you have a day where you are highly physically active, you may experience a lot of tiredness the next day, emotionally or physically. Take your time to recover, whether that means sleeping in, staying in, or just taking it easy for a few days. Don't push yourself too hard, and don't beat yourself up for relaxing. Not everybody can go at 100% all the time!

46. CHRONICALLY ILL PEOPLE ARE NOT LAZY

Sometimes, you won't be able to get out of bed. Sometimes, you'll have long stretches of time where you can barely function. During these times, you may have a tendency to think of yourself as lazy. But remember: your body requires more rest than a person without chronic illness. Listening to your body and giving it the time it needs to recover does not make you lazy. Do what you can on a day-to-day basis, and treat yourself with kindness no matter how productive you are.

47. DON'T LET OTHERS PATRONIZE YOU

There may be a tendency for others to call you "brave" or "inspirational" when you open up about your chronic illness journey, even if your intention was not to garner sympathy or admiration. But the fact that so many people miss when they call someone else "brave" or "inspirational" for just living their lives is… that they are just living their lives! People with chronic illness do not exist to "inspire" healthy people or make others feel better about themselves.

If you find that people in your life tend to treat you in this way, you can handle this in a number of ways. If you are close, try to explain why being called "brave" or "inspirational" can be hurtful. You are just trying to live your life, just like anyone else. You don't want to be held up on some chronic illness pedestal. If they are understanding, they will listen and make an effort to change the way they talk to you. However, if they are not so understanding, don't be afraid to cut them out of your life, or at the very least minimize your interactions with them. If you make posts about your chronic illness journey, you can hide those posts from particular people in your settings. This may reduce the number of times they can call you "brave" or "inspirational" – and you can get a much needed break from all that condescension.

48. YOUR RELATIONSHIPS WITH OTHERS MAY CHANGE

Throughout your chronic illness journey, you may discover who your true friends are. This can be a painful process, but ultimately, you want people in your life that will be understanding and supportive towards you in your healthcare journey. Healthy connections can greatly improve the quality of your life. So, to ensure that the people around you are the best support system you can have, there are a few things you should keep in mind.

Cutting off toxic people can be hard to do, but it is a necessary practice for everyone to learn, whether or not they are chronically ill. If you find your friends getting frustrated when you have to prioritize your health over hanging out with them, or they think you are exaggerating your illness in any way, these are not positive influences to have in your life and can be very draining to you in the long run. Even if someone is not particularly toxic, but is simply exhausting to be around – maybe they love to go on long runs that just are not possible for you anymore, or they enjoy big social gatherings that exhaust you by the end of the day – try to limit your interactions with them. You can certainly still be friends even if you tone down your relationship a bit.

If your friends are truly supportive of you in your chronic illness journey, they will have to adapt in your relationship with them if they still want you in your life. Friends and loved ones can either be the greatest source of comfort and assistance, or they could be your biggest downfall and drain of your energy. Be selective in the friends that you choose

and in the relationships you foster. You will thank
yourself for it in the end.

49. COME TO TERMS WITH THE FACT THAT YOU MAY NEVER BE "CURED"

Chronic illnesses are called chronic for a reason -
they can last for years, and potentially your entire life.
It can feel so daunting to think of how long you may
be dealing with your disease, and you may even feel
afraid of the complications that may arise as a result
of your illness. For example, my condition makes me
more susceptible to certain diseases, and can also
affect my ability to have children. These are fears I
have had to deal with since my diagnosis, and they
were certainly very difficult to come to terms with.

However, just because I may deal with these
diseases and complications in the future, and just
because I may always be living with my illnesses,
nothing is guaranteed. I may find that I never contract
any of the illnesses that are often associated with my
disease, and that I can indeed have children if I want.
Even if the worst case scenario happens, though, I
have realized that I will still be myself. I will find a

way to work through it. Even if I didn't have my chronic illnesses, I would still eventually contract some disease or health issue in my life, just like anyone else. And I will find a way to get treatment and still find time to enjoy my life, just like anyone else.

So, even though I might never be illness free, it is not something that is constantly on my mind. Most days, I am simply enjoying life and going through my routine just like anyone else might, maybe with a few extra complications. And that may be the way it is forever for me, or it may not. It's simply a journey I have to travel and see where it takes me.

50. DON'T MAKE THE MISTAKE OF THINKING THAT YOUR LIFE IS OVER

People with chronic illnesses live happy, fulfilling lives all around the globe. While chronic illnesses certainly affect your quality of life, sometimes on a day-to-day, debilitating basis, this does not mean that they define who you are. You still have your passions, your pet peeves, your likes and dislikes, your hobbies, your dreams – these are things that illness can't take away from you. There are fundamental parts of you that no illness can touch, whether they be physical or mental illnesses.

All human beings have value and have a purpose in being here. Being chronically ill is just another puzzle piece to add to the mix that is you; it is not the only defining factor. You will still be able to do things you enjoy, spend time with the people you love, and find meaning in your life. And though there are not many guarantees in a journey with chronic illness, that is one I can make for certain.

50 Things to Know

i

OTHER HELPFUL RESOURCES

i

READ OTHER

50 THINGS TO KNOW

BOOKS

50 Things to Know

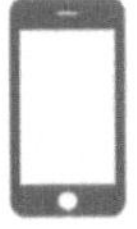

Website: 50thingstoknow.com

Facebook: facebook.com/50thingstoknow

Pinterest: pinterest.com/lbrennec

YouTube: youtube.com/user/50ThingsToKnow

Twitter: twitter.com/50ttk

Mailing List: Join the 50 Things to Know Mailing List to Learn About New Releases

50 Things to Know

50 Things to Know

Please leave your honest review of this book on Amazon and Goodreads. We appreciate your positive and constructive feedback. Thank you.